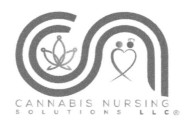

Dedication:

Madisyn and Maci, my M&M's, you are my why.

The reason why I have spiraled into my purpose.

May your purpose become clear to you as you move through life.

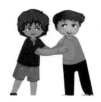

ASA'S

MEDICINE

By Ashley Wynn-Grimes

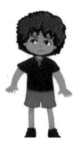

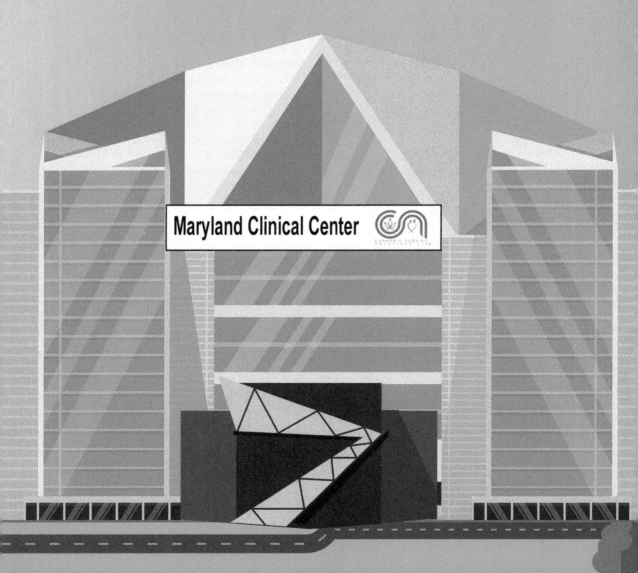

Asa and his family moved to Maryland so he could get a special treatment with really smart doctors over the summer.

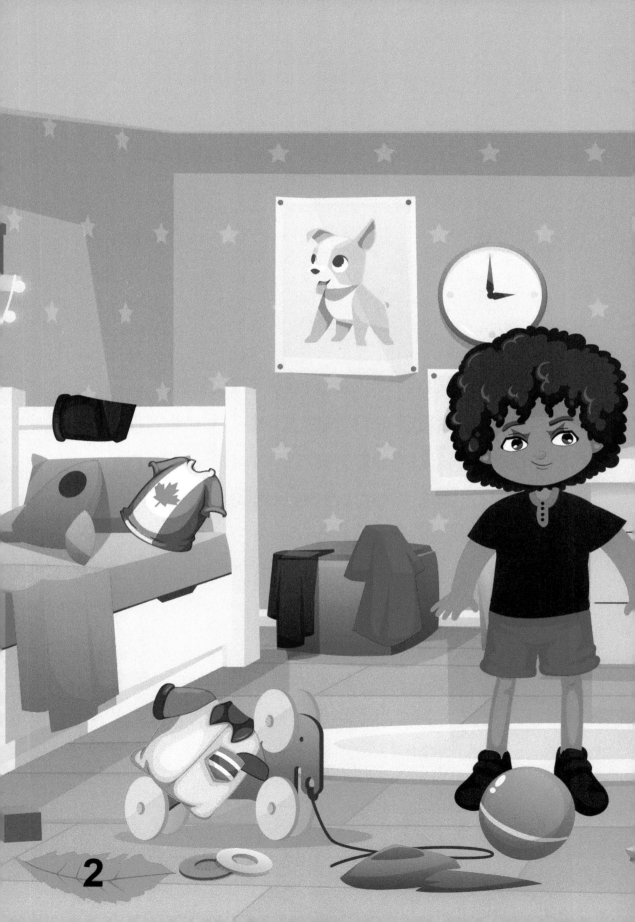

2

The night before the first day of third grade he began wondering if he would fit in.

What if they do not like his clothes, or the way he spoke?

What if they are mean to him?

What if he doesn't know the lessons and the kids laugh?

Will he have friends? What do they do at recess?

3

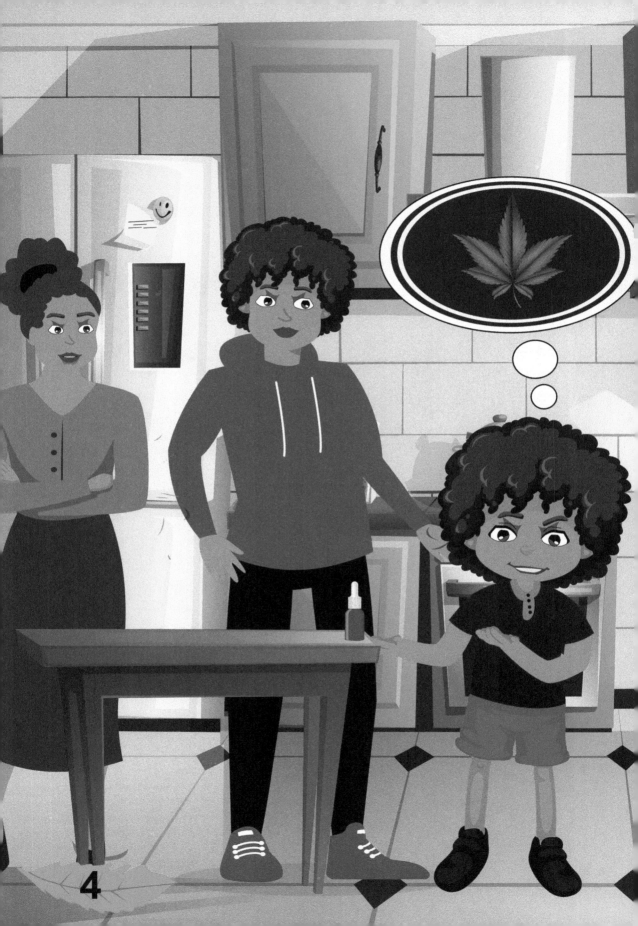

4

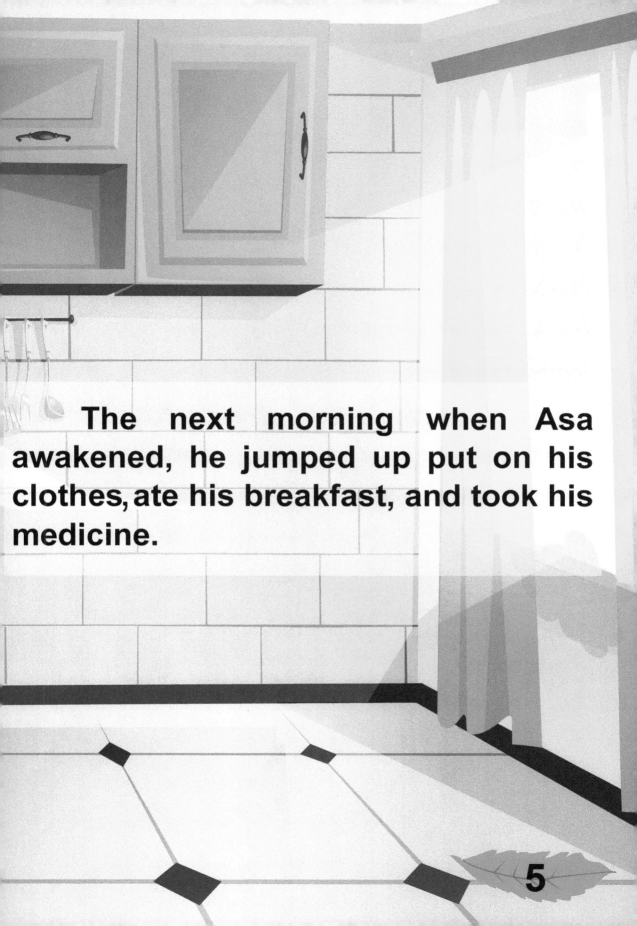

The next morning when Asa awakened, he jumped up put on his clothes, ate his breakfast, and took his medicine.

5

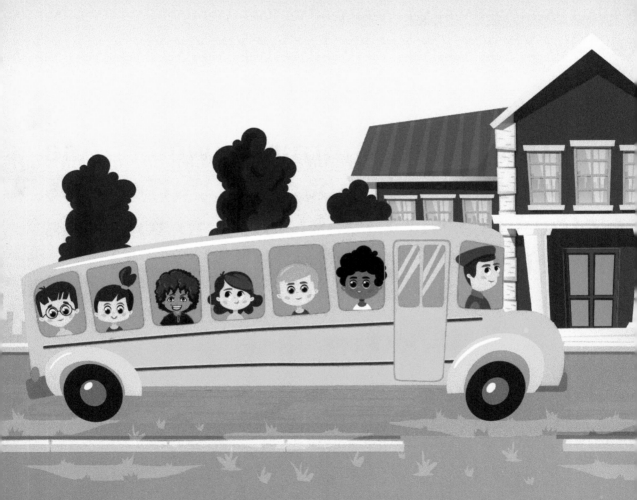

6

... And rode the school bus to school.

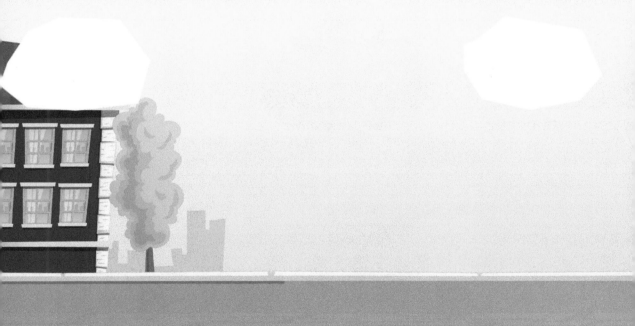

8

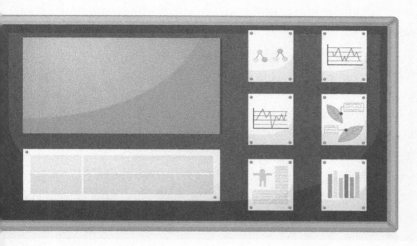

When he arrived, everyone was very excited to meet him. He was greeted by his new teacher, Mrs. Eliza.
The children crowded around him to greet Asa too.

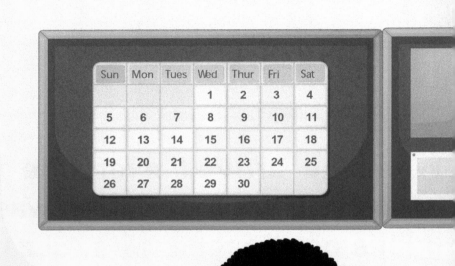

Sun	Mon	Tues	Wed	Thur	Fri	Sat
			1	2	3	4
5	6	7	8	9	10	11
12	13	14	15	16	17	18
19	20	21	22	23	24	25
26	27	28	29	30		

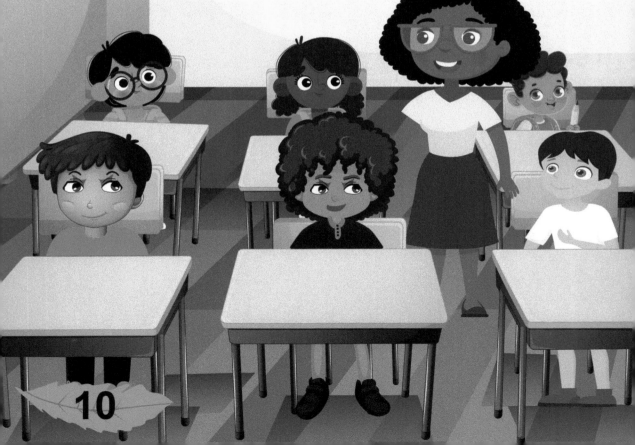

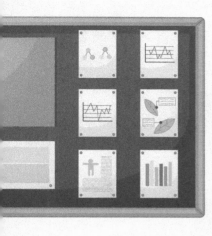

It was time to begin class and everyone sat down to learn.
Then Mrs. Eliza showed the students where everything was in the class and began with instruction.
Asa was excited that he was starting exactly where he left off with in second grade and he knew all the answers!

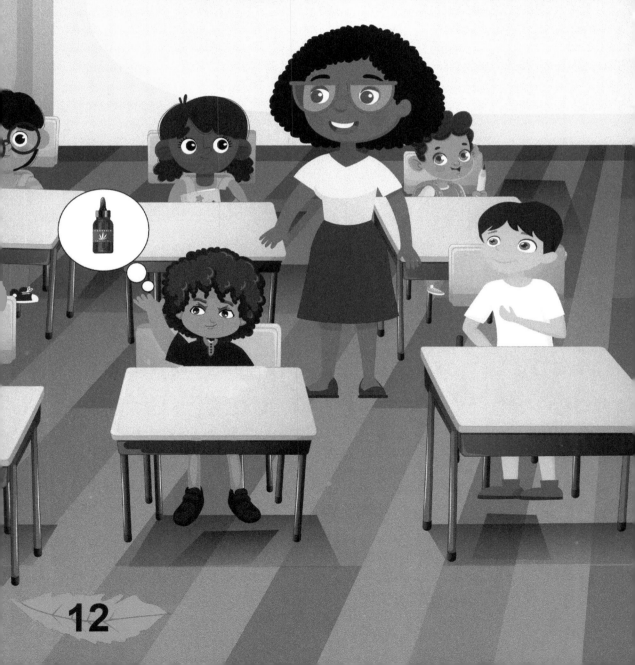

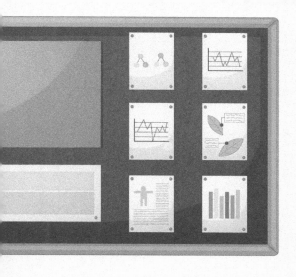

At noon it was time to take the next dose of Asa's medicine.
So he raises his hand to let Mrs. Eliza know. "Mrs Eliza, it's time for me to take my medical cannabis, can I go to the nurse's office?"

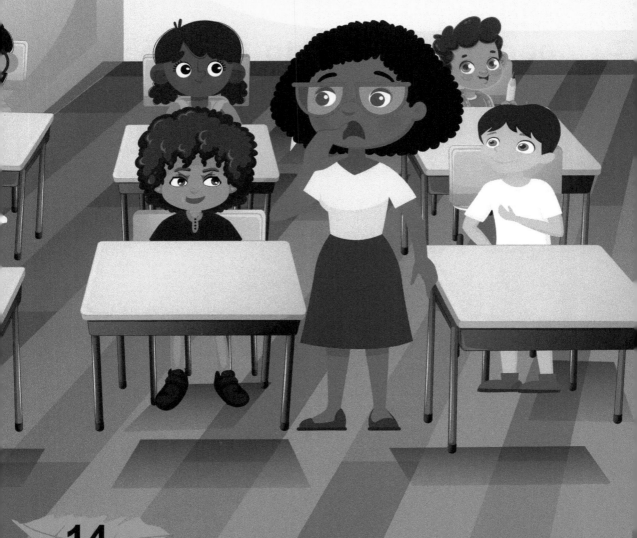

Sun	Mon	Tues	Wed	Thur	Fri	Sat
			1	2	3	4
5	6	7	8	9	10	11
12	13	14	15	16	17	18
19	20	21	22	23	24	25
26	27	28	29	30		

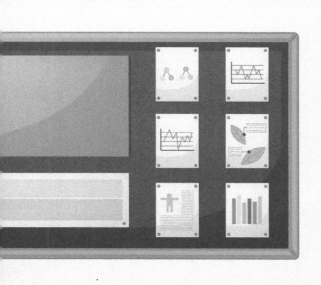

Madelynn asks, "What is medical cannabis?"…

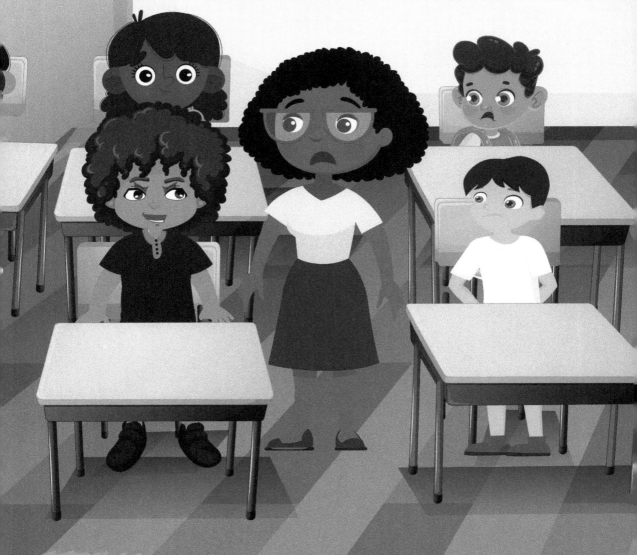

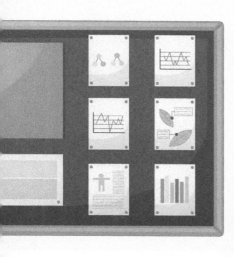

Asa responds proudly, "It's my medicine! I have to take it 3 times a day so I can do everything in the day. Without it I cannot eat and I get really sleepy. At first, my dad had to go to so many 'meetings' so I could take my medicine. I am not sure why, but people didn't like my medicine.

He was so exhausted from telling people about how important it is for me to take my medicine.

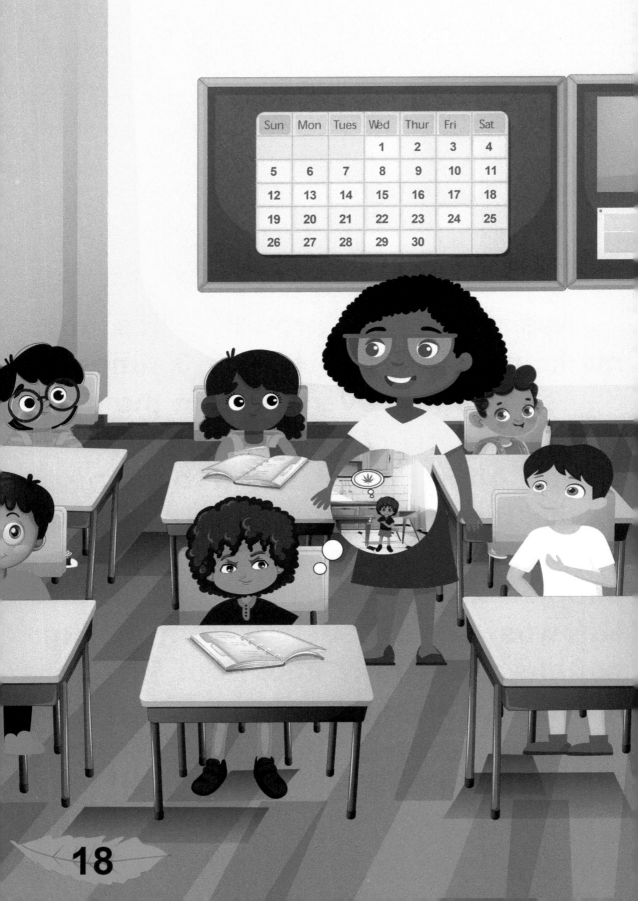

18

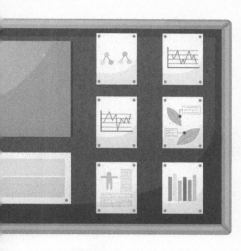

But now no one fights with him anymore about it.

I just take my medicine 3 times a day and I can play and learn all day!

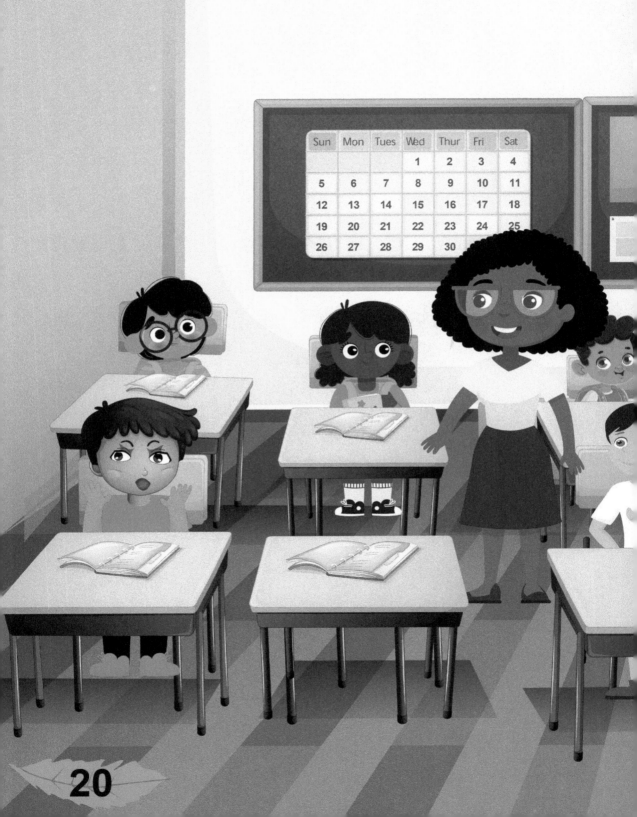

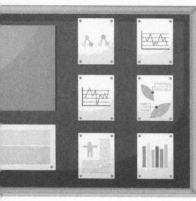

Rio says, as Asa walks out, "My mom says marijuana is bad for you! You are a drug user!!"

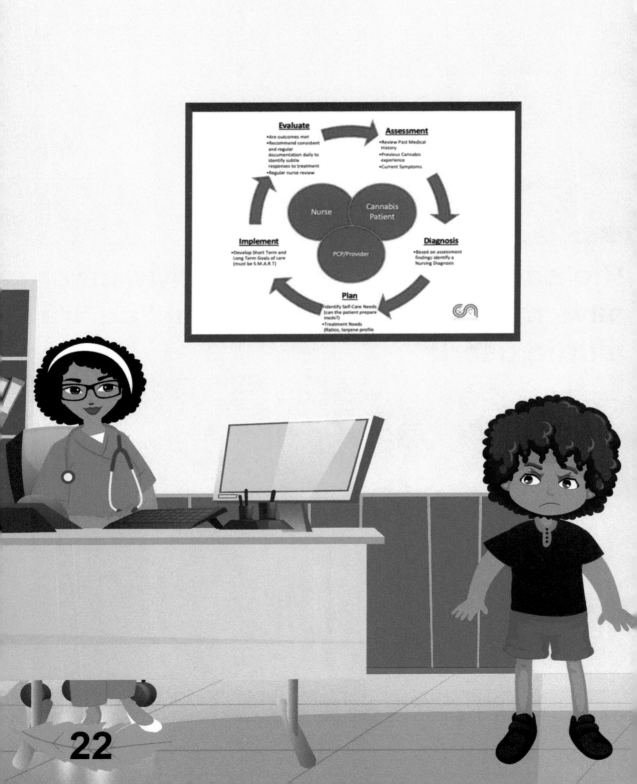

Hurt, Asa continues out the room to the nurse's office to take his medical cannabis and explains to the nurse what happened.

Nurse Ashley explains to Asa, "It is ok and we will teach them about your medicine. Your medicine has a long history where people learned to dislike medical cannabis and there will always be people who do not like that your medicine helps you, so it is our job to teach our friends about your medicine so they can understand."

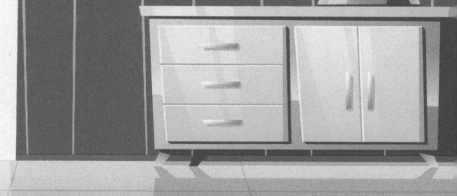

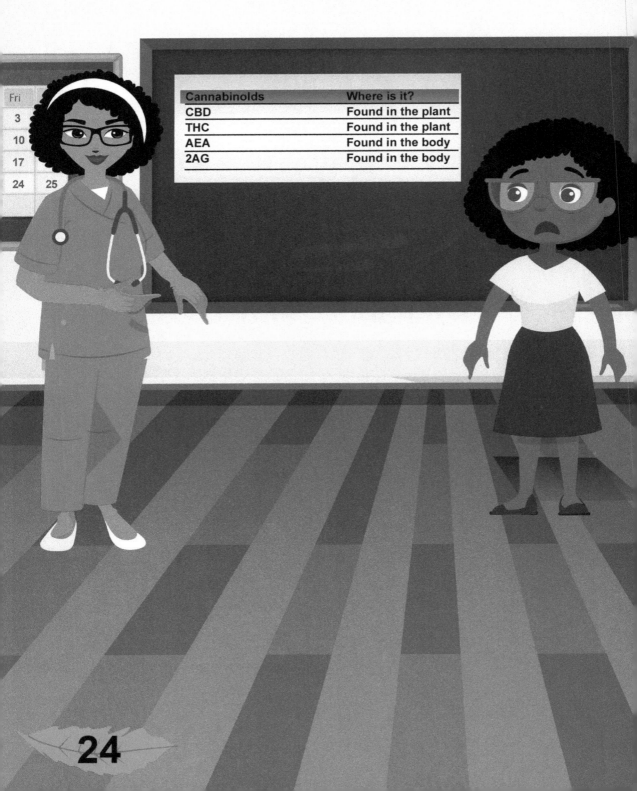

Nurse Ashley walks Asa back to class to discuss his medicine.

"Good Afternoon, I wanted to tell the class about medical cannabis.

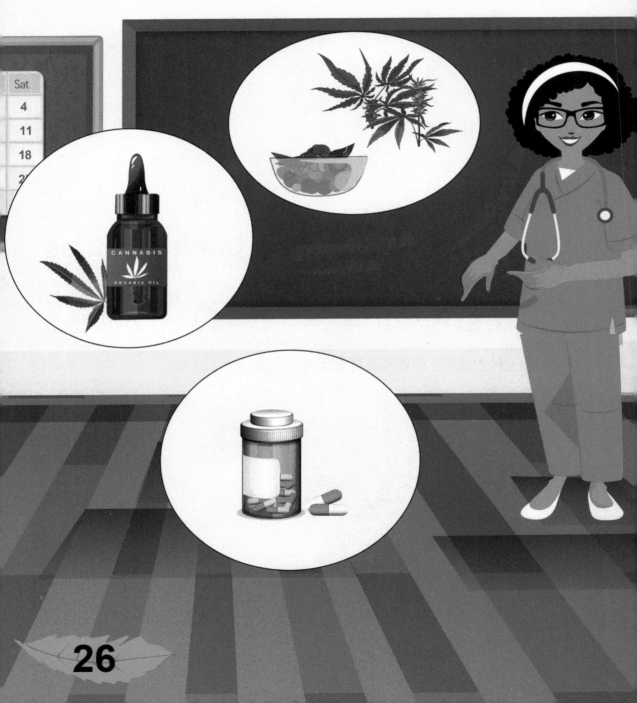

Medical cannabis is a dried flower that can be cooked and transformed to many things, but Asa uses droplets. He puts two drops under his tongue each time it's time for him to take his dose.

The two drops are perfect for his body and contain the perfect amount of cannabinoids and terpenes for him.

Since everyone is different, not everyone will need the same amount even if they have the same obstacles to overcome.

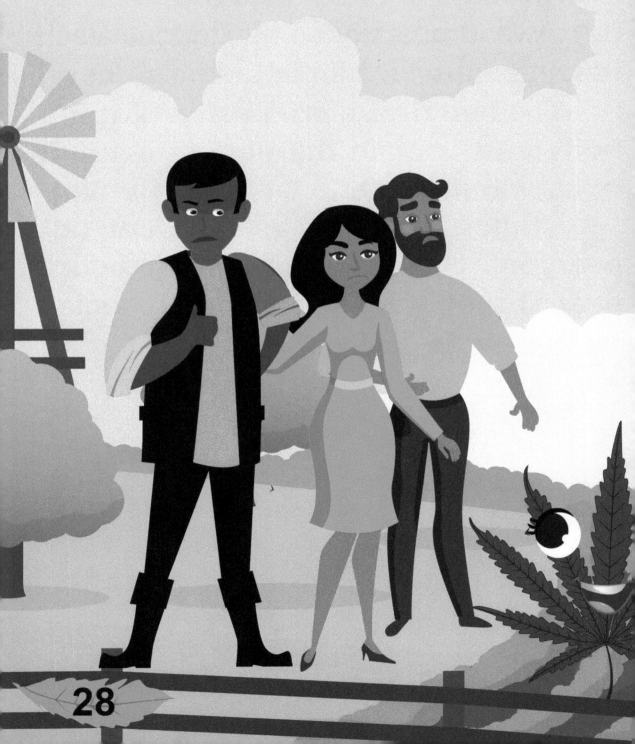

28

The reason why people do not like medical cannabis is because grownups did not study the plant   thoroughly enough to learn about all of the benefits it offers.

They thought that Cannabis was bad for the body and called it unkind names like marijuana, pot, devil's lettuce or weed.

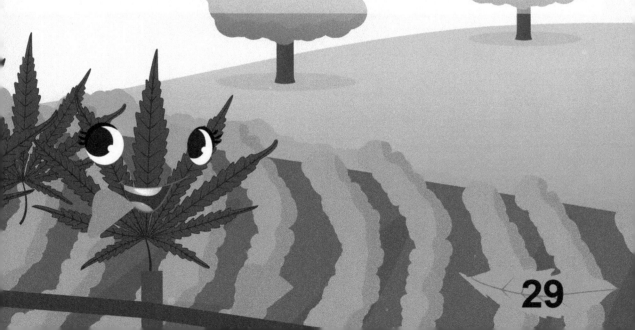

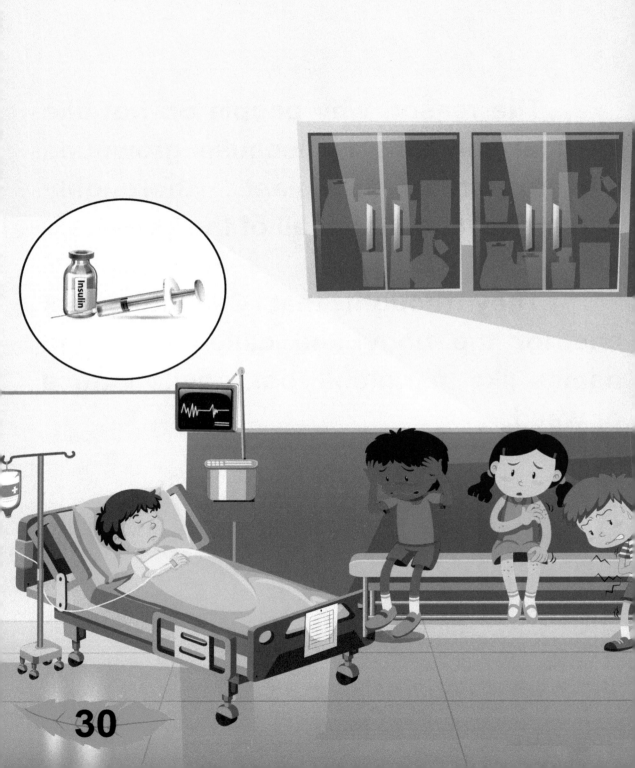

There are many of you who take medications regularly.
You have inhalers for your breathing problems, and insulin for high sugar. This is no different. Asa has gone to doctors to prescribe his medicine just like you did.

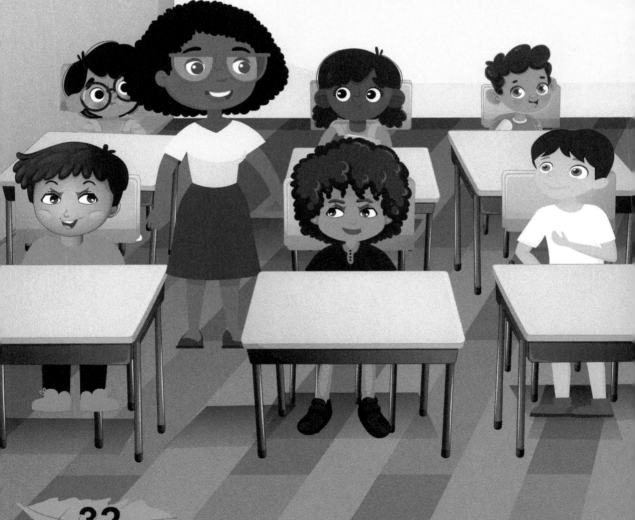

Sun	Mon	Tues	Wed	Thur	Fri	Sat
			1	2	3	4
5	6	7	8	9	10	11
12	13	14	15	16	17	18
19	20	21	22	23	24	25
26	27	28	29	30		

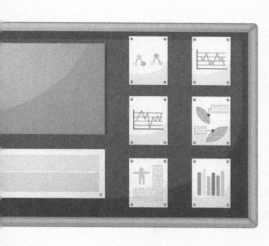

   Does anyone have any more questions?
No, ok have a great day!"

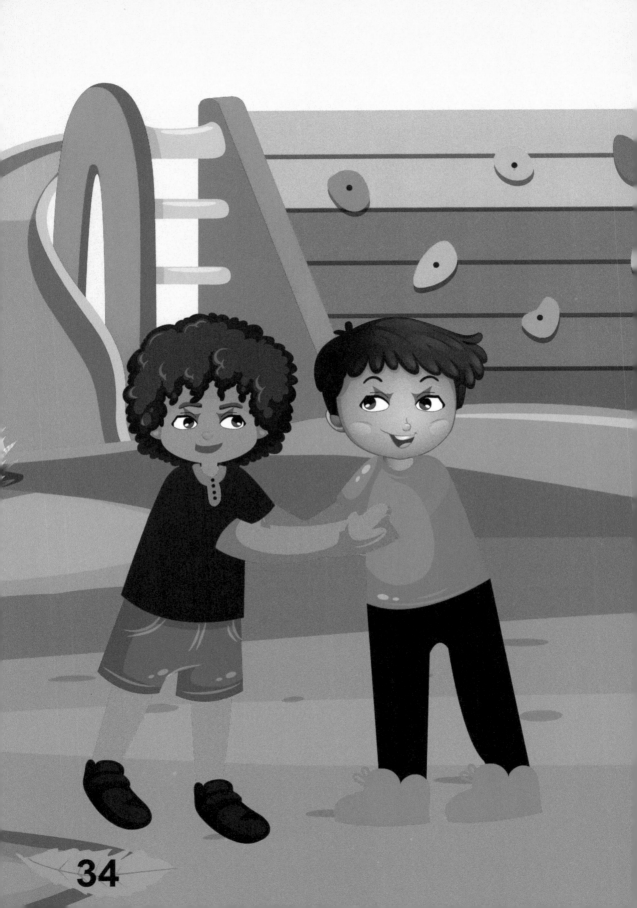

34

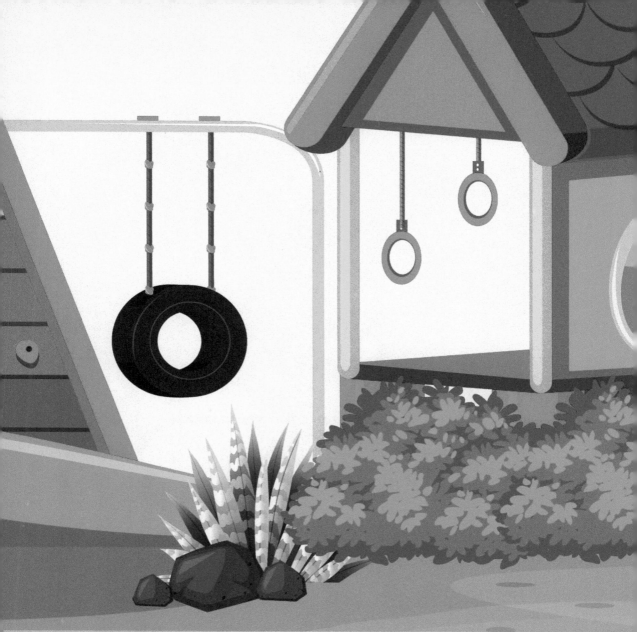

"I did not mean to hurt your feelings. I wasn't trying to be mean. Now I know that you are just like me!"

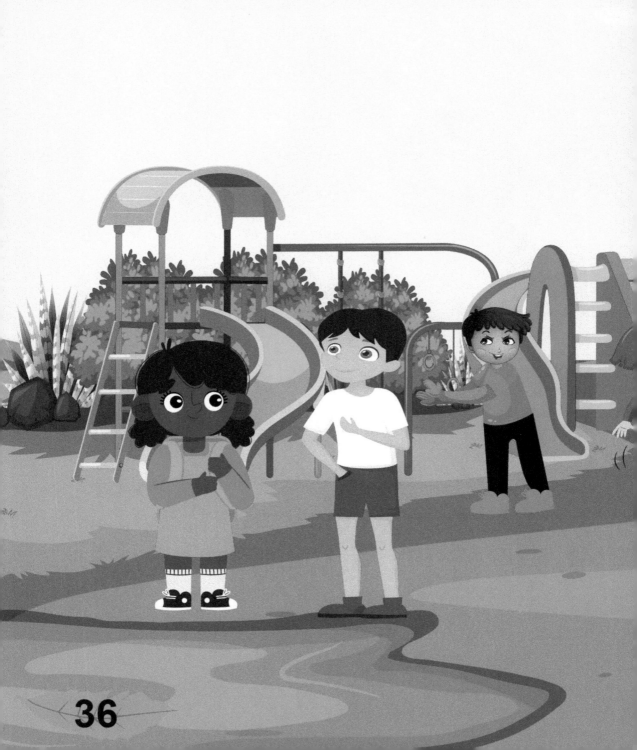

36

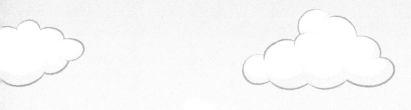

To Asa's relief recess was just like it was when he was in the second grade.

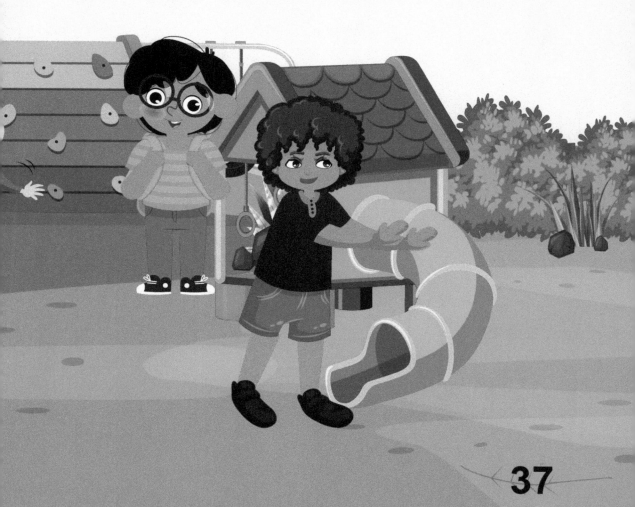

37

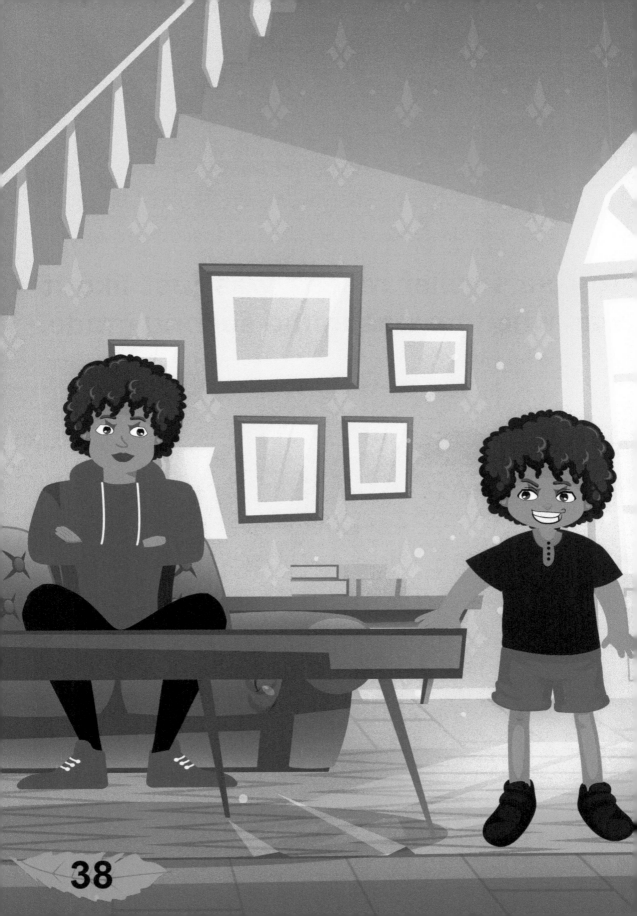

After school he came home to tell his dad how great his day was. He said, "The children were very nice and I taught them something too!!!"

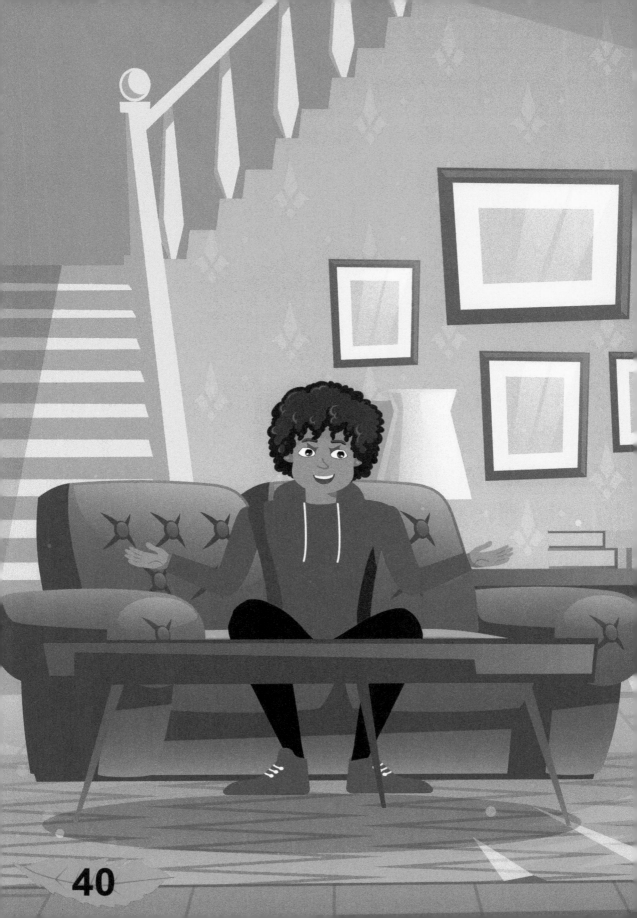

40

Asa's dad said, "Oh really? What did you teach them?"

Asa told his dad, "Everyone is different and has different needs, which really means we are all the same!"

As the popularity of cannabis medicine grows, so will the need for factual information and medical equality. This book was created as a stepping stone into beginning the journey of understanding cannabis medicine.

Please share with family, friends, neighbors and colleagues.
Thank you for your support,
Cannabis Nursing Solutions